A SHORT BOOK ABOUT LASTING LONGER

Step-by-Step Basics for the Management of Premature Ejaculation

by

Robert W. Birch, Ph.D.
ACS Certified Sexologist

A SHORT BOOK ABOUT LASTING LONGER:
Step- by- Step Basics for the Management of Premature Ejaculation

© 2007   Revised 2009   Robert W. Birch, Ph.D.

ISBN 10   1449523234
ISBN 13   9781449523237

PEC Publishing®
www.oralcaress.com

In memory of two pioneers
in the field of Sex Therapy

Helen Kaplan Singer, M.D.
&
Harold Lief, M.D.

TABLE OF CONTENTS

GOING SOLO

A FIRST TIME STRATEGY

A Rapid Ejaculation Self Assessment
begins on Page 53. Complete this questionnaire
now and then again after following through
with the recommendations that are laid out
in this step-by-step guide.

INTRODUCTION

Expectations

A lot of men and their partners wish they were innately able to prolong their passionate sexual encounters, vigorously thrusting in rambunctious intercourse for an hour or more. However, most men are incapable of such an impressive sexual marathon and many come to orgasm quite rapidly and, at times, unexpectedly. This early and abrupt ejaculation is often a source of profound disappointment to the men and their partners, often resulting in damage to the relationship and to the more fragile male egos. In fact, lack of ejaculatory control or *premature ejaculation* has been "officially" labeled as a *sexual dysfunction* and is the number one sexual complaint among men under the age of fifty. To understand this concern we should begin with the questions, "What is premature ejaculation?" and "Just how fast is too fast?"

Contributing Factors

I need at this point to state my preference to refer to the reaching of orgasm quickly as *rapid ejaculation*, rather than using the official label *premature ejaculation*. I believe that the word *rapid* is less pejorative, more accurate, and more easily defined. *Premature* implies an arrival before the usual or proper time, as in *premature* birth. To be premature is to be too early and that's not particularly good. On the other hand, *rapid* simply means *fast*. If you are in a foot race and you start prematurely, you are likely to be penalized but if, on the other hand, you start rapidly, you are just quick. I will agree, however, that there is a distinct advantage to starting a race quickly, while there is a distinct disadvantage to ending a sexual encounter within a matter of a few strokes.

It would seem, however, that there is not just one type of male rapid climax, but rather a wide range of ejaculatory concerns. There are a number of men who will ejaculate within seconds, often at the slightest touch and always prior to penetration. There are other men who are able to receive prolonged oral and manual stimulation without ejaculating, but once intercourse begins they will ejaculate intra-vaginally within a minute.

There are some men who report having been quick to ejaculate from their very first sexual encounter and remain so, but there are also those who report having been quick only during early sexual encounters and then somehow gaining control as the relationship progressed. Some men are perplexed by the fact they ejaculate rapidly with one woman, but not another. Some men claim they had been able to prolong intercourse over a number of years until suddenly and inexplicably losing control, while other lucky fellows seem never ever to have been bothered by an untimely ejaculation, while others slow down over time. It appears obvious, therefore, that there is not just one type of ejaculatory pattern, and even for each man his speed to orgasm might change from time to time or partner to partner.

There are a variety of factors that influence just how quickly a man will ejaculate, and age is one of these. A younger the man is likely to ejaculate more quickly than an older male. American comedian Joan Rivers once quipped, "I've stopped dating young men because of the game they play . . . One, Two, Three . . . Ready or not, here I come."

The intensity of the man's passion is another factor, as the more excited he is, the quicker he is likely to ejaculate, and related to this, the more novel and excited the partner, the greater the tendency to orgasm rapidly. Another variable is the frequency of a man's sexual release, and the longer the time period since his last ejaculation, the greater his inability to control. It is as though the internal pressure builds over time, and when the pressure is greatest, the release valve opens with very little provocation. The longer the internal build up of sexual energy, the less stimulation required.

It is also obvious that the more active and rapid the thrusting, the sooner the man is likely to reach the *point of ejaculatory inevitability* - that dreaded point of no return. Furthermore, it seems clear that the more worried or anxious the man, the shorter his fuse. In summary then, the man at greatest risk of ejaculating quickly is the young man who is with a hot new partner after a long dry spell and is both excited and nervous as he penetrates and thrusts wildly into a responsive and novel partner.

Some medications have been known to slow some men down, but this is a side-effect. Unlike the pills for men with erection problems, there is no pill that specifically targets the ejaculatory reflex.

"Normal" Endurance

You might now be wondering, "Just what is *normal* or *typical* male sexual endurance?" Let's first, however, consider the question, "What is *natural*?" In nature the purpose of sex is purely *procreation*, and this process commences with the mounting of a receptive female, quick pelvic thrust and the deposit of sperm deep in the vagina, independent of the time it takes to do so (or, for that matter, the partner's satisfaction). Intercourse is simply the means to the end – the deposit of sperm. Our primate cousins, the apes, chimps and monkeys, complete the act in a matter of seconds. As human beings, however, intercourse is most often for *recreation*, and typically great pains are taken to prevent actual conception.

Sex for humans is an expression of love, an avenue for the sharing of intimacy, a unique form of communication, a delightful source of sensual fun, and much more – and we have a certain emotional investment in being good at it! As human beings, there is more involved than in sex just our genitals. We make love also with our minds.

However, it does appear *natural* for a human male, like his primate cousins, to move the sexual activities progressively toward vaginal intercourse, to rejoice in the successful penetration, to thrust rapidly once in and, all too often, to ejaculate quickly in the completion of the seed-planting cycle. Mother Nature seems to be whispering into a man's ear, "Plant that seed and plant it deep, but be quick about it!" As you read on you will learn of some tricks that can be played on Mother Nature, who would have us get it up, get it in, get it off and get it out.

This brings us to the question of normalcy. When it comes to the ability to delay ejaculation, what is *normal* for the human male? I contend that it is quite normal for men, at the biological level, to feel the compelling urge to penetrate with an urgent desire to ejaculate quickly. At the same time, however, for a number of emotional reasons men typically experience the psychological need to prolong the pleasurable sexual connection. It can be assumed that female apes have never experienced orgasm and the male ape, having planted his seed, is unconcerned. The male ape does not care about his mate's sexual satisfaction, but we humans very much care about the fulfillment our partner's sexual needs.

Let us now consider the question of "What is *typical?*" Although reported averages vary a bit from study to study, it would appear safe to state that the *average* healthy male under the age of thirty, when engaged in steady vaginal thrusting, will most likely ejaculate in from two to four minutes (some reports state one to three minutes) . . . certainly not fifteen or more as many men often expect. The nature of sex works against our human wish to be able to last longer during sexual activity. Unfortunately, wishing often precipitates an even faster ejaculation.

To attempt to identify the *proper* time for an ejaculation to occur is a subjective venture. Who should decide when the time is proper – the man, his partner, the author of the sex manual on the bed stand? Some writers have assumed that the proper time for a male to ejaculate is either as or after his partner has reached her orgasm. With such an assumption, *premature ejaculation* has in the past been defined in terms of the percentage of times the man would ejaculate during intercourse before his partner could. This definition is actually quite useless, as we now know that the majority of women are <u>not</u> orgasmic with penile-vaginal intercourse alone. If as many as sixty-five percent of women are unable to orgasm during intercourse, a man could be able to thrust steadily for four hours with some women and still, by the old definition, be labeled a *premature ejaculator* (and his partner would likely end up unfulfilled and quite sore). If this same man were to go off and find another woman who was quickly and easily orgasmic during intercourse, he would lose the diagnosis. Therefore, it makes no sense whatsoever for a diagnosis of a male sexual dysfunction to be dependent, not on the man's duration, but on his partner's ability to orgasm during a coital encounter.

Another question I would pose is whether a quick male orgasmic response should even be labeled a *dysfunction*? A rapid climactic explosion by a woman, although atypical, would surely not be labeled a problem! Rapid orgasm is common among men and seems to be a natural condition that serves Mother Nature's procreative intent, requiring only that the man get it up, get it in, and plant his seed. As humans, however, we want to enjoy sexual union for more than occasional procreation. We want to be able to experience the intimate bonding, share the erotic pleasure and be thought of as a competent lover . . . all of which seems to demand the ability to postpone an ejaculation, as the male climax typically ends his erection and drains his energy to continue.

Trust that I will tell how a man can learn to improve his ejaculatory control, but I do wonder if we have been calling a natural function a dysfunction because our heads are wanting something other than what is hard wired into our bodies? If a large percentage of men ejaculate more rapidly than they think they should, if the average young and highly excited male ejaculates uncontrollably within about two minutes of continual penile stimulation, if Mother Nature's prime purpose for sex has been met, and if traditional sex therapy has not been particularly effective in effecting a lifelong "cure," how can we call it a dysfunction? A concern? Yes. A challenge? Probably. A disappointment? Usually, but a dysfunction? I think not.

Re-examining Expectations

Bare with me now, for I am <u>not</u> going to tell you that you must accept your hair trigger and live with it. God forbid that we should be stuck with always ending before our partners can even get started. However, I do want to emphasize the point that we are dealing with both an animal drive and a human expectation. Expectations are important and influence our perception of our reality. For a moment consider the couple in your neighborhood who last night spent a romantic evening snuggled together on their couch watching a video and eating pizza. They teased and fondled sensually, anticipating an intimate encounter that would top off their evening. After the video and following their showers, the woman put on soft music and the man lit candles. Once in bed, the two began to play. This was not *foreplay*, but was *for play*. They were in no hurry, they made no demands and they had no expectations other than to share the experience of each erotic moment as it unfolded. There was a lot of manual stimulation for the woman, and as the man caressed her skin, he spoke softly of how sensual he found her naked body and whispered of the pleasure he found in giving her pleasure. She did not avoid touching him, but she purposefully kept her caresses brief, having learned of his hair-trigger threshold.

In due time the man moved to the oral stimulation of his partner that for her, and many other women, is a great source of pleasure. For him the cunnilingus was an intimate act of giving. After about fifteen minutes of skillful finger play and cunnilingus, during which he built her almost to her climax, but then backed off, only to start building again. This teasing technique built the intensity of her arousal and the woman was pushed over the brink and experienced her orgasm (or orgasms as the case may be). As she settled down from her climactic high, her patient partner mounted, thrust hard and deep, and ejaculated explosively in lest than sixty seconds. They then snuggled together, still coupled, mutually enjoying the afterglow of a loving encounter, each pleased with the pleasure given and the pleasure received. This man ejaculated rapidly, but did not consider himself dysfunctional, nor did his grateful partner. The concept of dysfunction is inappropriate here, as each couple must define what is uniquely good, right and satisfying for them.

We will argue, however, that many men would not be happy with only sixty seconds of vaginal containment, and there are certainly many women who would also enjoy prolonged intercourse – some to the point of their own orgasm. It is obvious, therefore, that a man's ability to prolong intercourse is a problem if he says it is a problem, and it is a problem if his partner says it is a problem, and it does not take a consensus between the two to cause one or both psychological distress.

Potions and Pills

Men have tried many things to slow themselves down. Makers of the desensitizing creams have made fortunes because men believe if they can numb the head of their penises they will last longer. However, most men are disappointed with these overprice creams, as the extensive wiring for the ejaculatory reflex is much more complicated than just those superficial nerve endings around the end of a relatively short extension of the total neurological system. Someone once said that our largest sex organ is not between our legs, but rather between our ears, although there is a lot of very complicated neurology between the end of a penis and the pleasure center of a man's brain.

In recent years, some physicians have begun to "treat" rapid ejaculation by prescribing medications that were found to have ejaculatory retardation as a side-effect. However, as a behavioral scientist I have had a problem with the prescribing of a medication for its side-effects. Even if such medication would work (and it often does not), it will not "cure" a quick trigger. If the drug's side-effect does help, but nothing about a man's ejaculatory control is actually altered, will the man be willing to take it for the rest of his sexual life? In relying on a magic pill, albeit an expensive prescription drug, a man will never really learn to manage his ejaculatory process.

Condoms might help. However, I have talked with men who have been well prepared with a fresh supply of rubbers, but have in their excitement ejaculated when putting one on! Now that's really a bummer! One should always, of course, wear a condom to prevent the exchange of a sexually transmitted disease when with a new partner. Sex is fun, but not worth dying for. Also, in a long-term committed relationship, fresh and properly fitted condoms are an effective contraceptive device when wanting to avoid a pregnancy. However, wearing one just to delay ejaculation might prove more trouble than it's worth, but if a man wants to try this, the non-lubricated condoms are recommended. With a lubricated condom the penis slides a bit inside of it, which is why some men claim then feel more with a lubricated one than with a dry one.

Pathologizing a Natural Process

Unfortunately, much effort by well-intended sex therapists has been wasted, for many of my colleagues have not understood the dynamics of the natural ejaculatory response nor the important learning components of gaining better management of this complicated process. In part, the difficulty has been with the viewing by professionals of rapid ejaculation as a pathological condition, rather than a natural one. Calling it a dysfunction is essentially the perception of a natural process as an unnatural illness. In the medical model of thinking, if there is an illness, there is then hopefully a "cure." Thus we find many self-help books promising a cure in from four to eight weeks! If it is a natural and fairly typical response, what is there to cure?

I was not surprised to learn that a three-year follow-up study had shown that a significant number of the men thought to have been "cured," ended up right back where they started from before beginning treatment for their rapid ejaculation. Something is missing in the mechanic "prescription" of behavioral homework, given with the promise that faithful compliance, once completed it will produce a lasting lifelong remedy. Just doing the prescribed exercises will not change anything if something is not also being learned in the process that will be good forever. In other words, simply going through the physical act of a prescribed exercise will not lead to lifelong improvement, unless the man understands and remembers exactly what it is he must be attending to in that process.

It is most likely true that some men are just more sensitive than others. There is no "cure" for what is just another of the multitude of individual hard-wired differences we find among people. However, I had mentioned earlier two very common features of men who consistently ejaculate rapidly: High sexual excitement and high psychological anxiety. These are psychological influences that can be modified, along with some physical arrangements, that must be changed in order for a man to slow his natural progression toward ejaculation.

La La Land

When super excited, a man falls under the spell of Mother Nature and enters an euphoric altered state of consciousness. I have playfully called this euphoric start of awareness, "La La Land." In La La Land the man is overwhelmed with desire and his mind is focused only on the exquisite sensations he is feeling and the erotic fantasies he is experiencing. When caught up in this state, the man is essentially on automatic pilot and is on the short cut to his point of ejaculatory inevitability.

If a man is to learn an effective strategy for managing his ejaculatory response, he must not allow himself to become overly excited and become lost in that wonderful state of La La Land. Yes, ejaculatory control will cost a man something, for he cannot get totally caught up in his crazy-wild passion without dashing uncontrollably toward that point of ejaculatory inevitability. Increasing the frequency of ejaculation, either with a partner or through self-stimulation can help. Also staying relaxed both in mind and body is very important, and I will be saying a lot about that later.

The Role of Anxiety

We will need to consider the role of frequency and the need for physical relaxation. The other common feature of rapid ejaculators that demands our attention is mental anxiety. Anxiety has interesting, and at times devastating, physical effects on a man's sexual performance. If the anxiety is overwhelming, he will fail to achieve an erection or, if he has one, he will most likely lose it. This is the "performance anxiety" that is often the only cause of an erectile disorder. High anxiety is a form of panic and the physical reaction to it is as if Mother Nature is frantically yelling, "Sabertooth Tiger! Sabertooth Tiger! Forget about sex and run for your life!" With a lower level of anxiety, however, Mother Nature leans close and whispers, "There might possibly be a tiger close by, but it's OK to finish what you started . . . just be darn quick about it."

COUPLES' HOMEWORK ASSIGNMENTS

First a Short Story

Despite what I have said about how traditional sex therapy is often ineffective in "cure" a rapid response, there is value in the recommended behavioral homework when the focus is placed on what should be learned in the process and not just on doing the mechanics. There is no cure, but there is hope. There is nothing quick, easy or permanent when it comes to learning the strategy for lifelong management of the ejaculatory process. It takes time and a commitment.

Before beginning to lay out some helpful behavioral and cognitive homework, I want to tell a story that I have told many times. I call it: *The Plight of the Eager Young Fireman.*

On his 11th birthday Billy's father, a fireman, gave Billy a bright red fire truck. The boy loved the feel of it as he pushed it across the floor and was excited by the fantasy of racing to a fire and quickly extinguishing the flames. He dreamed of someday being a real fireman, just like his dad. He waited impatiently for high school graduation and hurriedly made application for admission to the city's firefighter's academy. His lifelong dream was answered when he was accepted into the training.

Bill was enthusiastic about the practice drills and continued to be quite excited by the thought of rushing to a real fire and hurriedly putting it out. Learning was good, practice was fine, and fantasy was exciting, but Bill was eager to get to the real thing. He yearned for the feeling of the heat he knew to be possible only with the actual experience.

Bill graduated from the academy with high honors. On his very first day in the station, a call came in and he was on the truck racing to the blaze. As he got close to the fire, he could feel the heat. The sights, the sounds and the smells were incredibly exciting and before he even thought about it, his ladder was up.

Bill, hose in hand, raced to the foot of the extended ladder and climbed toward the top. Suddenly he was falling! "Oh shit!" he muttered, "I've gone over the top!" He was embarrassed that he had not anticipated the last rung of the ladder and that he had fallen before he was able to extinguish the flames that had excited him so. He promised himself that he would do better the next time, but felt some anxiety as he anticipated his next opportunity to prove himself.

It was not long before he was again called upon to perform the task he had yearned for since his youth. Again he raced up the ladder and again he failed to anticipate the final rung. Once more he was muttering an "Oh shit!" as he flew over the top and plummeted down the other side. Bill began to feel even more embarrassed, and it seemed that the harder he tried, the more nervous he grew – and the worse his control became.

Repeatedly he would race up the ladder and invariably he would fly over the top before realizing he was even close. It didn't help seeing the other guys performing well and hearing the praise heaped upon them for having stayed so well and for successfully having extinguished the flames. "Certainly," Bill thought, "I am as motivated as they are, if not more so. Surely," he reasoned, "this control should come naturally to the son of a fireman." He knew he had the same passions as his father, but could never remember his dad saying anything about falling prematurely over the top.

One day Bill saw a beauty of a fire. He felt the heat more intensely than ever before. He knew there were spectators and he knew he was expected to perform well. It was obvious that his performance would be compared with that of the other fireman, and he really wanted to do his best. The ladder was up and extended to its full length. Bill jumped to the task.

Gritting his teeth tightly and clinging firmly to his hose, Bill raced for the top. A moan of disappointment arose from the spectators as Bill flew wildly over the top of the ladder. Flying through the air on his way down he could be heard to exclaim, "Oh shit, I've done it again!"

Bill was sitting on the curb, head in his hands, when a veteran fireman approached. "What's wrong, young fellow?" the older man asked Bill, who was now looking very dejected.

"I love the excitement of being a fireman," Bill responded, "but I never can stay on the ladder long enough to get the job finished. I can get my hose up quickly, but before it can put out the fire, I go over the top. It's been happening every time, and now I'm afraid to even start."

The older man was silent, recalling his own early embarrassments when he too was new at putting out fires. It was Bill who broke the silence. Obviously still wanting to look good, Bill stated, "I don't know what I'm doing wrong. I get very excited about squelching the flames and I want to do the very best job I can, so I run up the ladder as quickly as I can.

But I just can't seem to stop myself from falling over the last rung and I don't have the energy to run back up again for another try."

After considering Bill's dilemma, the more experienced man observed, "It would seem to me that in your excitement you forget to watch where you are going, and by the time you reach the top rung it's too late to stop! The next time you head up that ladder, slow down, look ahead, and keep track of where you are. When you see that you're approaching the point of no return, stop before you get there!"

Getting Started

Relaxation and a non-demand atmosphere are essential to the learning process, so I will outline a series of steps intended to help both man and woman "get out of their heads" and into their senses – to become more aware of all the internal signals that can be missed in La La Land. Remember that being *sensual* means to be employing all your senses as you interact with your partner in the following encounters. Enjoy her with your visual sense as you survey her nude body. Smell the back of her neck and elsewhere to enjoy her with your olfactory sense.

As you caress her, "be in your finger tips" so you are able to appreciate the feel of her warmth and softness as your tactile sense tells you of the textures her skin. Lick the inside of her elbows (an erogenous area for many women) as you experience her body through your sense of taste and listen with your auditory sense for the sound of her breathing or the gentle moans that might emerge as she relaxes with your loving caress.

SENSATE FOCUS - STEP ONE

Focus on Sensations

It was the pioneers in sex therapy, William Masters and Virginia Johnson, who had initially brought the idea of *sensate focus* to our attention. Specifically, these pioneer sex researchers introduced sensate focus as a valuable tool in treating a variety of male and female sexual dysfunctions. This behavioral "homework" is surprisingly uncomplicated and the premature ejaculator and his partner need not do the entire program as outlined by Masters and Johnson. For our purposes, we will talk of *sensate focus* as the creation of a situation within which a couple can learn to *focus on sensations.* Others have used the term "non-demand pleasuring," but I like to think of it as "intimate sensual caress."

As a first step we will look at the value of focusing on sensations while engaged in non-demand <u>non-sexual</u> pleasuring. This provides an excellent opportunity to study your own broad range of sensations and learn more about those of your partner.

You and your partner must first agree to put intercourse off limits and to avoid touching each others breasts or genitals. Yes, you read correctly. **Call a moratorium on intercourse and no playing with erogenous parts!**

If there has been a problem with getting too excited and too tense, and if the goal and fear have centered on having "successful" intercourse, the most logical way to begin to reduce performance anxiety is to first work on changing the goal. It is easier to relax if there are no expectations other than the exchange of sensual touch. Intercourse will not forever be off limits, but to start let's focus on the process and not the goal.

In this non-demand atmosphere, with intercourse temporarily forbidden, you can allow yourself to leisurely practice giving and receiving non-sexual pleasure. In the process of decreasing performance pressures, many men with unreliable erections find a more consistent genital response when not feeling the demand to get it up! Neither is there the expectation that the man will keep it up, if intercourse is not allowed and genitals are off limits, and one quickly learns that the world will not end if an erection falls! During this step it is okay if you get an erection, it is okay if you lose an erection, and it is okay if there is no erection at all. This is a "fail-safe" concept of sexuality. With the focus on having fun and not on having intercourse, all kinds of new feelings will emerge.

For some, this will be a brand-new experience, having in the past touched only as foreplay. If *foreplay* is touch that precedes intercourse, this touch is just *for play*. The goal is not prolonged intercourse, the goal is to discover the process of mental and physical relaxation and to find joy in the sensual exchange of mutual intimate caress.

Plan to set aside an hour, at least twice a week. The more often you are intimate with your partner the better, just as long as it is with mutual agreement, stays within the limits and is relaxing. Once a week is perhaps too infrequent, but may be practical in terms of your schedules. I am realistic about busy schedules, demands of work or school, and, for some, the responsibilities some have as a parents.

With busy schedules you may even need to write a reminder on your calendar. You may protest that this does not allow for spontaneous encounters, so let me suggest that you think of it as "scheduling your spontaneity." Many couples in having to schedule their "dates" find ways to make time available that they had not realized they had. Also, you can and should always be spontaneous with your <u>non-sexual</u> touch between your scheduled "dates." Do not put your affection on a schedule!

Plan to do the non-sexual sensate focus for about two weeks. You may feel like you are going to explode, and in fact you might. If it happens, it happens and that is okay, although let this be a reminder of how easily you reach your threshold. If you really cannot get together more than once a week, and need to deal with your own sense of urgency, perform the solo exercises described later to fill in the gaps. The goal of the solo self-stimulation is not to ejaculate as many times as possible during a week, but rather to find a frequency that feels very natural for you, a frequency that matches your level of libido. Ejaculating less than that frequency may mean you will have a tougher time relaxing and staying under control with your partner.

Schedule your hour at a time which is well <u>before</u> your usual bed time, for when it is time to sleep and you are tired, you will most likely hurry through your homework. Schedule it earlier and within the time you have scheduled, take quick showers (perhaps together) so you are each feeling fresh. Light scented candles and put on some nice music (preferably something you cannot sing along with). Have some warm massage oil at the bedside, or handy beside you on the floor if that is where you prefer to be. Massage oils are often sold in store specializing in bath supplies and skin creams. If you can find pure unscented coconut oil, that also works well when heated. In selecting a massage oil, chose one that is not quickly absorbed or becomes sticky.

To begin, lie together naked and just cuddle. Lie quietly, breath deeply and begin to relax. Avoid passionate kissing and remember, breasts and genitals are off limits for now. **The goal is to relax, not to arouse**. Once you feel relaxed, take turns giving and receiving a soft sensual massage, being erotic, but not sexual. As you are caressing your partner, experience the texture of her skin and the warmth of her body with your fingertips. Focus on this <u>process</u> of receiving pleasure through giving it. Try to remain relaxed, as **this is one of the most important things that you must learn in managing your ejaculatory response.** Do not rub your penis against your partner or on the bed, and stay relaxed. No cheating!

Do not worry about performance. Do not worry about lasting. For now, with sexual touch off limits, all you need to focus on is the joy of sensual caress – both the giving and the receiving.

Caress your partner's back, her buns and the back of her legs. When she turns over, do her shoulders and arms, tummy and legs, but avoid her breasts and genitals. If in the process of caressing your partner you feel that you are about to ejaculate, stop, get up and walk around the room. Come back once you feel under control. Do the same while your partner is caressing you. Study your sensations and watch for those bodily signals that tell you where you are in terms of your relaxation and in terms of your excitement.

Find that balance where you can relax, feel pleasure in giving and receiving and remain in control. If you lose control and slip into La La Land, don't beat yourself up, but pay closer attention the next time. Mother Nature will hurry you along if you are not careful. Like the young fireman, you have to learn to recognize where you are on the ladder.

Trade off who gets to receive first so that every other session you give first and on alternate nights you receive first. Both as giver and as receiver, focus on relaxation and on the pleasure of giving pleasure. Talk of what feels good and learn from each other how each likes to be touched.

Discover new erogenous zones, such as the feet and the smooth hollows behind knees and inside elbows where the nerve endings reside close to the surface of the skin. Really tune in on your feelings, both as giver and as receiver, and stay playful.

The Importance of Effective Feedback

I believe most couples do not touch enough, do not talk enough, and too often fall into the pattern of touching only as the silent somber prelude to sex. Someone once said, "It is easier to do sex than it is to talk about it." Take this opportunity to give feedback, to learn what feels good, and to learn to put your thoughts and feelings into words. Because of this opportunity to work on verbal communication, I recommend that you spend at least two weeks with the playful non-sexual sensate focus -- longer if you could only get together once during each week.

Be positive in your exchange of information. It is much more effective to say something like, "That feels OK, but I really love it when you touch me a little firmer," as opposed to, "You never touch me the way I like." It might help to think about giving *I statements*, rather than *you statements*. "I like it when you touch that spot," versus "You never seem to touch me where I like it best." Practice giving positive directions and practice listening carefully to the feedback offered by your partner.

Deciding When to Move On

Try your best to do this first step of the sensate focus non-sexual caress for at least two weeks, at least twice per week. **Do not progress to the next step if you feel anxious (nervous) or tense.** You will only set yourself up for more disappointment if you hurry too quickly through the learning steps! Be sure that you and your partner are both able to relax and that you and she will both be comfortable once you being including genitals in the homework of subsequent steps.

If you and your partner are a couple that has been avoiding each other, you may not be ready to jump right into the homework that is more sexual. Stay with this non-sexual step until both of you are absolutely ready to move on. Do not rush in the process, for you have a lifetime to master this, and it might take some time to become comfortable with each other if there is a history of avoidance.

If because of emotional distance in your relationship you do need this non-sexual time to grow close again, stay with this first nonsexual step. In the meantime, to deal with your own sexual drive and to begin learning some of the principles of ejaculatory control, you should begin the solo practice described later in this book.

Although this sensate focus is not intended to directly effect your rapid ejaculation, learning to relax is an essential element and in sexual encounters it is important that you are able to distinguish when you are tense and when you are not. When relaxed, the exchange of this sensual touch is likely to trigger some response. Remember, in doing the non-sexual homework it is okay if you feel sexually excited. The important thing is to stay in touch with the level of your arousal and, if it begins to escalate, to back off from what you are doing. Remember the young fireman who could not anticipate the end of his ladder and, as a result, would fall over the top. You need to be learning where you are on your ladder. If you've gone into La La Land, you are in danger of losing control. Separate from each other for a brief cooling off period. Talk a bit or get up and walk around. Return to the sensual touch once you feel you are back under good control.

I do worry about suggesting fourteen days or more without sexual release, and I think sex therapy often fails because moratoriums are presented as unbreakable. If you need to spend time becoming relaxed, working on communication and reestablishing feelings of intimacy, you will find that filling any gaps with masturbation might be essential to your ongoing management. A section on masturbation is presented in a later section.

If you wish, once a week and <u>separate</u> from this sensual homework, you can have intercourse or bring each other to orgasm in other ways, but you must feel relaxed before beginning. Since you are not working directly on ejaculatory control at this stage, **agree not to worry about stay power and the duration of intercourse**. Pleasure each other and just let the orgasms happen, being sure of course that your partner gets her turn to orgasm also. Do not take advantage of the invitation, however, to pursue orgasmic release and neglect your sensate focus exercises. Let an orgasm be the reward for being good students and for faithfully doing your "prescribed" sensual homework, and stick to your schedule. Do not decide midstream that a non-sexual date should be an opportunity for a quickie! Either do the agreed upon sensual homework, or agree <u>in advance</u> that it will be okay to have a quickie.

Discovering the pleasures of taking (or making) time to give and receive sensual massage allows you to return to it at any time in the future. Be sure to "stay in touch" as you move on to the more sexual assignments. In a long term relationship, sharing intimate and sensual love is far more important than making genital and sexual intercourse. Learn now the pleasures of erotic caress and develop skills that will be valued for a lifetime!

SENSATE FOCUS - STEP TWO

Moving On

It is important to feel relaxed and to feel some semblance of control, albeit without sexual stimulation, before moving onto the second step. This step is the transition between working on relaxation and beginning the work on gaining better management of your automatic flight into La La Land. Continue to schedule your sessions, that one of my client couples called their "lube jobs" given the amount of massage oil they were lovingly and lavishly smearing on each other's naked body.

For this second step, it is essential that the two of you focus in on the shared verbal feedback. By now, if you are relaxed, you should be feeling enough control that you can "specialize" in giving sensual pleasure to your partner. Take time now to more fully explore her body, enjoying every nook and cranny. Be generous in your giving, as soon she will be asked to give an equal amount of attention to you. **Yes, her breasts and genitals are now on limits, but do not dive for them!** With her help, become an expert on her total body. Let her words and sounds guide you. Explore your partner's body with your hands and with your mouth. Tell her how good she feels and tastes to you. Focus on an awareness of all your senses and the pleasures they bring into your awareness as you experience this sensual contact with your partner. As your hands explore her contour, visually enjoy her body while listening to her soft sounds, tasting her essence and smelling her feminine aroma. **Get in touch with all of your senses without the goal of intercourse!**

As you go through the homework that is coming up, always begin (or end) with a full body caress and erotic sex play for your partner. With orgasms coming on limits, I do suggest that you give to her first, as many men lose motivation after they have ejaculated. Noting this, Dr. David Schnarch, noted sex therapist, observed that women have orgasms, but men have "snorgasms!" Many women have already learned that if they want some special time, they had better get theirs before their man ejaculates, because once he has finished, it is his nap time!

It is important that your partner feels that you have an interest in her pleasure. She will be asked to give a lot in future exercises and it is important that she knows there will be something special in it for her. Now that her genitals are on limits, do not rush. A premature dive for the crotch is a turn off for most women! Move slowly from a sensual massage to a sexual caress. Remember, most women, once comfortable and relaxed, will respond best to direct clitoral stimulation. Ease up to the caress of this most sensitive "pleasure bud." Be careful if she has not already begun to lubricate, as this area is very sensitive. Rubbing a dry clitoris may prove more irritating than arousing. If lubrication is needed, use an artificial water-soluble sexual lubricant such as K-Y Jelly or Astroglide, and be gentle until her arousal builds.

If you have been using a massage lotion with a vegetable oil base, do not use that oil on your partner's genitals! As one can never be sure of what grows in massage oil, avoid the risk of causing a bladder or vaginal infection and keep these oils away from her genital area. Additionally, you should never use Vaseline on a woman's genitals nor as a lubricant for intercourse, as this petroleum base jelly will not mix with a woman's natural lubrication (her *transudate*) and may actually retard her production by clogging the pores from which her slippery wetness seeps.

Stay relaxed and do not lose track of where you are. Your partner will understand now if you have to stop or if you get up and move. However, always remember that if, as you are giving pleasure, you become so excited that you come when she does without being touched, do not beat yourself up and do not apologize! Read this as an indicate that you will need to increase the frequency of your sessions together or, in filling in the gaps, you might need to masturbate more often.

Step Two provides a wonderful opportunity to learn more about your partner's sexuality and to perfect your skills in arousing and satisfying her. In this erotic homework assignment you can practice giving sensual and sexual pleasure without having to worry about prolonging intercourse. Remember that intercourse is still off limits, but you may stimulate your partner orally if this is something you both enjoy. If this is already a mutually enjoyable activity or if you both would like to explore its potential, do not rush the *cunnilingus*. Ease into the oral caress and tease for a while. She'll appreciate the build up.

After you have followed your partner's directions and have fulfilled her desires, it will be your turn. You will be starting the *start/stop program* at this point, assuming that you are relaxed and feeling some sense of control. The start/stop program will be described a bit later.

Remember, if you happened to ejaculate just from the excitement of manually or orally caressing your partner, do not become upset and offer no apology. Rather, tell your partner of your great excitement in giving her pleasure and the enjoyment you felt as you came while pleasuring her. Recognize how sensitive your nervous system is and redouble your efforts to keep track of where you are as you progress toward that point of no return. Stay aware and know when you are slipping (or plunging) into La La Land.

That Tingly and About-to-Explode Feeling

Before going any further, I've got to mention something important! If you have ever experienced this *tingly about-to-explode sensation*, you will know exactly what I'm talking about. It comes on much quicker than slipping into La La Land and it is much more intense. It's an unmistakable, right-on-the-edge feeling, from the very start and you want to cry out, "Don't even breath on it!! It is that awareness that the lightest touch will instantaneously trigger an explosive orgasm! The penis feels electric and the man is ready to pop and he knows it! With some men this happens only during the earliest and most exciting encounters with a new partner (novelty is a powerful aphrodisiac), but with other men it happens on a more frequent and persistent basis. High anxiety and intense excitement have combined and the result feels irreversibly explosive!

There are two things you can do if this happens to you. You can just let'er rip or (my recommendation) you can get up, start moving and keep walking until that feeling begins to diminish. It will fade if you give it a few minutes. When some semblance of control returns, explain as best you can, get yourself settled down and go back to your play. In the Start/Stop exercises you will learn to better monitor your level of arousal and know when it is essential to slow down or stop.

START/STOP - STEP ONE

Learning Management

This is the first step of your control homework. With your partner, continue to schedule a realistic number of sessions per week, giving these sessions the time and priority that you had given the sensate focus exercises. In each episode, be sure that you pleasure your partner so that she will not feel neglected. For these two weeks of your stop/start training you will be pleasuring her as in Step Two of the sensual caress assignment described above, including breast and genital stimulation. As mentioned earlier, I recommend that men satisfy their partners while still highly motivated, and this usually means giving to her first.

When it is your turn to receive, lie down on your back and allow your body and mind to begin to relax. Your partner should begin touching you with non-demand sensual caresses, caressing your body in non-sexual ways as you continue to relax. As you relax, focus in on the feeling of your partner's hands on your body and of any sexual response to this. Some men will become quickly aroused even with non-sexual caress, while others will not. There is no right way to respond. However, if you become aware that your excitement is escalating too rapidly during this non-sexual touch, have your partner stop. Lie quietly until you feel you are back in control, and then signal her that she can once more caress you.

Once you feel completely relaxed, under good control, and fully aware of your body's internal signals, ask your partner to begin slowly caressing your penis with her dry hand. Imagine that you are starting at the foot of a ladder. As your partner moves from non-sexual touch to the stroking of your penis with her dry hand, you will no doubt experience yourself climbing that ladder quite quickly. Your focus must shift from the pleasurable sensation of her hand stroking your penis to where you are on that ladder. Concentrate on where you are in your climb. Keep close track and, as your excitement grows, imagine yourself ming higher and higher up that ladder, a rung or two at a time. It is your responsibility to keep yourself from falling over the top and, as the veteran fireman advised, you must look ahead in order to anticipate that point of no return (the point of ejaculatory inevitability). **To focus only on the erotic sensation in your penis is to stand dangerously close to the gates of La La Land, that altered state of consciousness where Mother Nature eagerly awaits you!**

Lie perfectly still! Do not move and do not tense your body. Keep your eyes closed and avoid any sexual thoughts or images. You need to be concentrating only on where you are on that ladder! When you are approaching the point of no return, tell your partner to stop. If you wait until you are there, it will be too late and you cannot afford to play brinkmanship with this fragile trigger. When you feel you are getting dangerously close to this point, your partner should stop stroking, let go of your penis and sit back. It might take a minute or more, but you should feel yourself level off and, in a few more moments, to begin descending that ladder. Do not instruct your partner to start again until you are absolutely sure that you are back under control and standing at the foot of that imaginary ladder. Once settled and back under control, signal that she can begin the stimulation again.

While at this step, sexual stimulation should be minimized. **No oral stimulation of your penis is allowed and your partner's hand must be dry. Even then, she should stroke slowly.** Remember (and remind her) that she should not be trying to bring you to orgasm, but rather needs to be providing the stimulation that will allow you to learn to better monitor your level of arousal.

You should not move a muscle while being stimulated, and do not allow your body to tense. Mother Nature wants you to move and wants you to tense. We want to fool her. It is best if you don't watch your partner's body as she pleasures you. Mother Nature has made men responsive to erotic visual stimulation. With your eyes closed and your mind devoid of erotica, mental contributions are minimized. Without any muscular feedback from your body, and without visual stimulation and mental imagery, it will be easier for you to focus on those inner indicators of your level of arousal. Being able to focus clearly will facilitate your learning to effectively monitor your level of excitement.

Start and stop five or six times in each session before allowing yourself to ejaculate and when you do, see if you can identify what it was you did to give yourself permission to go ahead and come. It is good to be learning how not to ejaculate, but also to learn to know how you let go so you can. There is a good chance that your partner, during this stage of the exercise, will also be learning about your body language as you progress toward your orgasm.

You might have noticed how your partner's body tenses as she approaches orgasm. This *hypertonicity* is more easily identified in women than in men, but guys also automatically tighten up a bit as they get close. In fact, many men and woman consciously tighten muscles to speed and intensify their orgasmic response.

I recommend that you stay at this stage of the stop-start procedure for no less than two weeks, but I always feel that staying longer at each step allows for better learning. Longer at each level is absolutely necessary for the men who come each time with the slightest touch. It is best not to rush any of these steps, as it is better to learn what you need to learn the first time through.

This homework should not be too frustrating, as with each session you will have the opportunity to bring your partner to orgasm and then to ejaculate with your partner's manual stimulation. Even though intercourse is off limits for now, you can still have fun exploring the various erotic avenues to bringing your partner to her climax. If she has a favorite toys or wants to try a new vibrator, this might be the time for her experimentation.

If you have not already done so, now would be a good time to explore your partner's G Spot. Insert two fingers, palm up and curl them, making the "come here" motion up behind her pubic bone. You might feel spongy tissue that seems to swell with stimulation, or feel nothing. She might feel pleasure, annoyance or nothing. Combine G Spot stimulation with cunnilingus. When between her legs orally stimulating her clitoris, insert your two fingers palm down, but once in you can turn your hand to caress up behind her pubic bone. You chin will be in your palm. Talk of how this feels. Does it add to the pleasure, distract from it or do nothing?

If to remain in some control, as you are being stimulated mentally and/or physically, you need to increase the frequency of your ejaculations beyond what is comfortable for your partner, fill the gaps with the solo practice described later in this book. Do not attempt to pressure your partner into a frequency greater than what she desires. It is far better to take care of the excess sexual energy yourself than to risk turning her off by pushing too hard.

START/STOP - STEP TWO

Adding Sensations

Continue to schedule your "dates," ideally working in two or three sessions per week. I am amazed by how others therapists have unrealistically advised couples to do their home-play every single night! That is usually not practical for most couples, and pressure to get it done with the prescribed frequency risks turning an otherwise fun exercise into work. In addition, if a couple does actually force a nightly practice ritual while practicing, they will not really have prepared themselves for their more typical and more widely spaced routine.

When you have made the time that fits best into your schedules, start sensually as before in previous sessions with some erotic play for your partner. Remember, if at any time your arousal suddenly begins to escalate or you have one of those tingly-and-about-to-explode experiences, stop everything and, if needed, get up and walk! Stay in touch with your feelings and, once settled, come back to bed.

Be sure to excite and satisfy your partner in the ways that she loves to be pleasured. Spoil her, and she'll surely return the favor! When it is your turn to receive, begin with some non-sexual caress and be sure you are feeling relaxed before inviting your partner to stimulate you sexually. When you are feeling relaxed and under control, your partner should stroke your penis with her dry hand until you have had to stop her two or three times.

Now your partner should begin manually stimulating you with a slippery lubricant of your choice -- warmed if possible. If she is comfortable with it, at this stage your partner can stimulate you orally. Regardless of the stimulation, manual or oral, you must keep track and you must stop her before reaching the last rung of that imaginary ladder. The use of a lubricant and the option of oral stimulation makes this step much more exciting than the last, so be careful. Do not play brinkmanship, as you will be risking an unplanned ejaculation. Stay relaxed and do not move. Do not fantasize and keep your eyes closed. Think of that ladder and stop your partner before it's too late. **Remember that it is better to stop ten strokes too soon than to stop one stroke too late!**

Within each episode, start and stop five or six times and do this home-play step for at least two weeks (if not longer). Do not rush things! As always, let your ability to relax and your growing awareness of internal signals be your guide when it comes to making the decision about moving on to the next step.

START/STOP - STEP THREE

Outercourse

Continue with your scheduling, but check with each other to be sure that neither of you are feeling pressured. It is absolutely essential that your playtime together remains fun and relaxing. Intimacy and caring remain top priority, with ejaculatory control somewhere down the list. Between the two of you, reaffirm that! Hopefully in working on the control, you have both been working on opening up your communication and have acquired a greater appreciation of the advantages of starting slowly with non-demand and non-sexual caress. Do not lose the desire and appreciation for sensuality as we move onto the more sexual levels.

Begin each scheduled session with an exchange of non-sexual caress and, as always, find out what you can do for your partner. When it is your turn to receive, get on your back again and relax! Nothing new here! Stay calm and do not move and do not tense. With eyes closed, experience your arousal as your partner, using a dry hand, manually caresses your penis. Keep track of where you are on the ladder and start and stop her two times.

Now she should stroke your penis briefly with a good safe water-soluble sexual lubricant. For this, good old inexpensive K-Y Jelly will do. After getting you good and slippery, your partner should straddle you, nestling down onto you so that your penis is between the lips of her genitals (her *vulva*). You are not to penetrate. With the artificial lubricant and any of her own, she should slide along the underside of your erection, sliding front to back, but without inserting your penis into her vagina. Intercourse must remain off limits, but this *outercourse* is perhaps the next best thing.

Sliding back and forth with plenty of lubrication should feel good to both of you, but you must continue to keep track and stop her when it begins feeling too good. Anticipate your point of ejaculatory inevitability and stop her before reaching it. Start and stop five or six times during these sessions, and repeat this step for three weeks. During the first week do not put your hands on your partner and keep your eyes closed. However, during the second of those weeks, open your eyes and put your hands on your partner's hips or thighs. Be careful and keep track, always ready to say "Stop," or if you are holding her hips, stop her non-verbally by locking your arms.

During this process, learn how to evaluate and monitor the impact of the stimulation you are getting through your eyes and your hands. Subtract this out as you near the point where you must stop, closing your eyes and removing your hands. If you feel your excitement level off, carefully ease a little closer to the point where you must stop. When you must stop her during the <u>first and second weeks</u>, she should lift up, breaking the contact between her vulva and your penis. Do not move! Feel yourself drop off the high level of excitement and, when you are sure you are back under control, invite her to sit and slide again.

<u>During the third week</u> I would like you to begin to ease more of the erotic aspects back into your awareness. Start with the visual, and then try adding a bit more tactile stimulation. If you feel under control, add some caressing of your partner's breasts during the outercourse. Keep close track of your progression – where are you on that ladder? Allow a little fantasy, but do not move and remain perfectly relaxed. Feel your partner's warm slippery vulva sliding over your penis, but go back to your monitoring, from time to time checking your position on that imaginary ladder. Stop your partner's movement only after you have tried decreasing your own inner stimulation (stopping the visual input, stopping the touch, etc.). If you feel your excitement level off, ease a little closer to that point of no return – but be very very careful!

During the first two weeks you had her lift up when you stopped her, but during this <u>third week</u> I would like you to see if you can settle yourself during each pause with your partner becoming motionless but maintaining genital contact with you. Begin adding to your verbal directions. Initially you just had two instructions – "start" and "stop." Now you can add "slow down," "easy," "don't move," and "lift up."

You can now have the option slowing her down, but you must stop if you sense you are rapidly heading into La La Land. Short of that, begin to practice changing the stimulation rather than terminating it. Feel the good feelings of that warm contact, but also keep track of your excitement level. Ease a little closer . . . slow her . . . stop her for a moment . . . take a short break as she sits quietly, warming your penis between the lips of her vulva. Keep track and see if you can level off at a high level of excitement and still feel some sense of control – but be very careful!

START/STOP - STEP FOUR

Exciting New Step

After three weeks of the outercourse homework, each week having added something more erotic, it is time to take the plunge . . . literally! After the usual non-demand start and the gentle exchange of sensual caress, and after taking turns with some mutual genital play (the start/stop variety for you), get on your back and relax. Your partner should now straddle you and, for a few moments, just sit on you with your penis resting between her outer vulvar lips. Experience the warmth of her genitals against your penis, visually appreciate what you can see of her body, and rest your hands on her thighs. At the same time, with that split-screen you have hopefully developed, monitor your level of excitement.

Once you feel settled, have your partner begin to slide, signaling her verbally or with your hands. Watch her body, feel the power of her pelvic movement during this outercourse and sense her warmth and wetness, but keep track. Getting too excited? Close your eyes, clear your mind, think of taxes! Slow her or stop her if necessary.

There are some sex therapists who would discourage your thinking of baseball scores or, my favorite, imagining a pending audit by the dreaded IRS. Those who would not approve of using mental diversion believe that this will distract from the monitoring of arousal, the only task a man should focus on. While this may be true at earlier stages of the home-play, by now I feel that a mental distraction can be quite helpful. Since it is natural for a man to conjure up erotic fantasies and explicit mental images, inserting a non-sexual *thought wedge* can disrupt this process. Wedge these non-sexual thoughts into the stream of sexual imagery just long enough to help slow things down. Start and stop several times. Do not hurry.

Once you are absolutely certain that you are relaxed and under good control, instruct your partner to lift up from your body and insert your erection into her vagina. Sitting astride you, she should guide your penis to her vaginal opening and slowly lower herself onto you. It is important that there has been sufficient play to arouse your partner, as the presence of her natural lubricant is essential for an effortless penetration. You should not move during any part of this, and your partner should also become completely motionless once she has lowered herself down onto you! Experience your excitement build with this wonderful feeling of warm, wet containment.

Should you ejaculate with the first engulfment of your penis, do not worry and do not apologize. This might happen the first time. After all, it has been several weeks since you were allowed this grand entry. If it is unavoidable this first time, just let'er rip and enjoy your ejaculating inside your partner. If this happens over several encounters, consider the possibility that you may need to increase the frequency of your joint encounters or of the masturbation that you have been using to fill any gaps. You might even need to back up in your homework, starting back at a level where you felt you had been able to stay in control. If, however, you find that you are able to maintain control with your partner mounted on top of you and your penis snuggled passively within her vagina, signal her to begin moving slowly. It is important that she leans forward, supporting herself with her arms, and that she stays in tight against you. Her movements should be a sliding from front to back, rather than riding up and down. There are three good reasons why I recommend this in-close front-to-back sliding. First, it is easier on your partner's legs if she can slide and does not have to bounce up and down.

Second, most women will discover (if they have not already done so) that they can get superb stimulation by staying in close and rubbing their clitoris against the base of the man's erection. When they lean forward, their hips rotate back and upward, and if a woman concentrates on what she is feeling, she is then able to mentally make contact with her clitoris and keep it rubbing against a firm surface.

The third reason has to do with that hardwired program – the one where Mother Nature says, "Thrust long and deep as you slide your sensitive penis its full length in and out between the walls of that warm and exquisitely slippery moist vagina." Remember, no one had to teach men how to thrust. If Nature has built in the male thrusting response, and if a man is getting some erotic feedback from his hip muscles, then the strategy is to resist what has been designed to work the fastest.

Relax as you lie flat on your back. Remain completely motionless as your partner slides. Since she is the one in motion, you receive no erotic *proprioceptive* feedback from the pelvic muscles you would be using if you were the one thrusting. Also, when your partner stays in tight against you, the stimulation provided by the tight muscles surrounding the opening of her vagina are staying at the base of your penis, not sliding up and down the full length of your penile shaft. While it feels good, this is not exactly what Mother Nature had in mind! Her procreative strategy is to have you thrust wildly.

Keep track of your escalation toward that point of no return. Let erotic visual and mental stimulation in, but wedge it out if you feel yourself racing toward the brink and need to settle yourself. Visually enjoy your partner's breasts as she hovers and moves over you, but close your eyes if it starts to become intense. Dare to move just a little, but keep your thrusting minimal and be ready to relax if you need to in order to calm yourself? Stay in touch with your feelings and with your level of excitement. *Ejaculatory control* is control, not a cure!

Beyond the Homework

Within each encounter, start and stop as many times as you wish, as you are no longer under strict homework requirements. Experiment with how long you can go without deciding it is time to ejaculate. Talk together about how you can keep the frequency of your encounters up as a way to maintain a manageable level of excitement. After several weeks as you begin to feel confident that you can read your body's signals and accurately monitor the level of your arousal, modify the stimulation to find ways to hover at a nice (but safe) level.

At this stage you can begin experimenting with new intercourse positions, but always remember that you must continue to monitor your level of arousal at all times. Also remember that fast thrusting with long strokes will move you rapidly toward your point of ejaculatory inevitability!

Therefore, regardless of your position, stay in close, be sure to thrust slowly and with shorter strokes than your biology would dictate. Do not let Mother Nature decide how you should make love!

GOING SOLO

Practicing Without a Partner

It is much easier to learn and maintain ejaculatory control when a man is in a stable relationship with a steady, understanding and responsive partner. But what about the fellow who is without a steady partner or whose partner is uncooperative. It is possible to work on control alone, but it is a bit like trying to learn to play golf during the winter by watching a video and putting golf balls across the livingroom carpet into a coffee cup. While alone, a man can perfect that skill, but when spring comes and he is out for the first time on a real course with a real friend, things are a lot different! The excitement is far greater, but so too is the pressure to perform well!

If you have no partner at all, do not avoid masturbation. As George Carlin once said, "Masturbation is making love with your best friend." There is no pressure and there is no critic to judge your endurance. Men vary in terms of the level of their sexual drive, so you must find and maintain the frequency that works best for you. However, this is not a competition! Every day is okay and once a week is okay! What is important is to discover your natural schedule and then maintain it.

You will know you are pushing your limits if you find

that you have to work in order to reach orgasm. The object is not to try to see how many times per week you can ejaculate, the object is to establish your own unique pattern. You will know that you are not masturbating enough if you feel "horny" for a couple days and ejaculate rapidly even when trying to work on your control.

Most men masturbate by "jacking off," the up and down stroking of the penile shaft with a hand. The sexual stimulation experienced is similar to the in and out stroking experienced during intercourse, although a man will typically grip his erection tighter than the grip of a woman's vagina and the stroking is often faster. This hard fast movement is why the practice is also referred to as "pounding your pud" and "beating your meat." At no time during the early attempts to maintain control, the stroking should not be hard and fast, as the solo participant at this point wants to come as close as possible to the experience of being inside a vagina. A vagina doesn't grip like a tight fist!

Men who have learned to masturbate in other ways (e.g., rubbing on their bed, using a vibrator, or stroking with an artificial vagina) should practice the first steps of the following exercises with the more traditional hand stroking. Go slow and take your time, remembering that you will not learn control overnight. An investment of time and a whole lot of patience is going to be required.

First Step in Going Solo

Set aside enough time to relax and quietly think about what you want to accomplish. Nothing within these steps should be rushed. Slow, easy and relaxed are the keywords.

Establish your own frequency based on your own level of recurring desire, and each time you masturbate do so without the use of a lubricant, without using visual stimulation, and without fantasizing. It should be obvious to you that these restrictions are intended to minimize the amount of mental and physical stimulation and maximize your ability to stay focused on your changing level of arousal. With a slow light strokes, do the Start/Stop technique described in the couple's homework section and within each episode start and stop a least five times before allowing yourself to ejaculated. Remember that you must monitor your level of excitement and stop the stimulation <u>prior</u> to reaching the point of ejaculatory inevitability. Get in touch with those inner signals, do not lose track of your progression and do not play brinkmanship with your trigger point.

Use this time to clearly identify what is happening within your body as your excitement builds, thinking of this like running up the rungs of that ladder. After starting and stopping the desired number of times, decide that you want to ejaculate. Make it a conscious decision and ease into it, experiencing fully that approach to your point of ejaculatory inevitability. Continue with the slow stroking until you orgasm. Did you experience what you did to maintain control as you anticipated that last rung of the ladder, and then what you did to let go and fly over the top? What was different when it was time to orgasm? Did you tense somewhere in your body? Did you automatically stroke harder or faster? Was it just more of the same stimulation, but with a psychological shift from monitoring your level of arousal to experiencing the erotic pleasure or calling up a hot fantasy? You must learn to identify what is going on before you will know how to bring yourself under control.

Repeat this first step on your own schedule for two or three weeks, or better yet until you are absolutely sure you have learned how to keep close tabs on what is happening. It is better to take too long practicing a step than it is to hurry ahead. Slow, easy and relaxed! If you feel that you are out of control at any point in the following steps, return to this dry hand approach and relearn how to control with limited stimulation. Then after two weeks of repeating this previous less exciting routine, move ahead again.

Second Step Going Solo

Stay relaxed! Do not attempt a practice session if you feel anxious or tense. Remember that anxiety has no place in your sex life, alone or with a partner.

Once you feel as though you have mastered the ability to predict and prevent your ejaculation with the dry hand start/stop program, add a lubricant. Some men find Vaseline works, some have used a soft margarine, while others might prefer K-Y Jelly. Whatever works! With water soluble lubricants, such as K-Y, it is wise to have a container of warm water handy. A little water added to the lubricate as it begins to feel gummy will bring the slipperiness back. Whatever your lubricant is, it is good to warm it if you can, wanting to begin to approach that warm slippery feeling of vaginal intercourse.

Avoid visual stimulation and fantasy during this second step. Stay relaxed and do not move anything but your hand. Remain motionless.

Do the lubricated start/stop on your usual schedule and again, within each episode start and stop five or six times before allowing yourself to ejaculate. Sense the difference between control and permission to "head for home." Practice this step for two or three weeks, or until you are absolutely sure that you are under control and can accurately track your inner progression. I will again remind you that there is no cure, only a strategy that must become a part of your sexual routine, alone or with a partner.

Third Step Going Solo

Are you feeling any anxiety? If so, postpone your sessions until you are feeling more mentally relaxed. Hopefully you are getting the message! **It is very important that you feel relaxed, both in your mind and in your body.**

Continue as before with the lubrication, but now begin adding visual stimulation, mental images and sexual fantasies. Continue with the start and stop formula as before, and continue to monitor your arousal even as you attempt to add more and more sexual stimulation. Keep the relaxation and remember not to move anything but your hand. Mother Nature wants you to thrust and would have you respond to the internal feedback from the muscles in your pelvis. Not moving and not tensing helps with control. Stay with your personal frequency and with each encounter, start and stop at least five times before allowing yourself to ejaculate.

Are you keeping track now? Can you sense the climbing of that ladder of excitement and anticipate the point of ejaculatory inevitability well before getting to it? Practice this step for two or three weeks, or until you are sure you are ready to move on.

Fourth Step Going Solo

Now you can become more creative with your self-stimulation. If you had an alternative approach to masturbation, try it now with the start/stop principle built in. Continue with the lubrication and try some new ones. Enrich your fantasies and bring in some new visual material. Try different positions, add some pelvic thrusting, buy a vibrating toy, or purchase one of those artificial vaginas or masturbation sleeves sold in the adult toy catalogs. Above all else, when increasing your arousal with added stimulation, keep track and start and stop at least five times before allowing yourself to ejaculate.

Fifth Step Going Solo

Continue now as in step four, but rather than stopping, slow your stroke and attempt to hover at a high state of arousal, but not so high that you flirt with that flash point. You are now experimenting with managing more arousal than in previous steps. Again I will remind you that you need to keep very close track of your excitement and, although trying to maintain control at a higher level, be careful! Remember the dangers of slipping into La La Land and allowing Mother Nature to have her way with you. Your goal is to stay aware and gain better management skills.

As you experience yourself approaching that point of inevitability, slow your stroke, look away from any stimulating visual material, stop any movement in your pelvis, relax any tension you feel and end any fantasy that you might have been having. Without stopping, minimize that stimulation and return to bare bones stuff as you feel yourself level off. Stop, however, if you feel you had ventured too close and are still about to lose control.

As you feel your excitement drop with decreased input, increase the combined stimulation again, slowing and/or stopping five or six times before letting go , and even then, ease into it! Are you aware of what you did to give yourself permission to let go?

A FIRST TIME STRATEGY

Coping with a New Relationship

As had been said, it is a lot easier to learn ejaculatory control with a steady partner than trying to learn it alone. A steady partner will know the rules of the start/stop program and the two of you would have talked about realistic expectations. With a brand-new relationship, however, there is no history of having worked on the concern together, and you will have no idea what is expected of you. Also, as we all know, new and novel relationships are bound to be more exciting and anxiety producing.

Unfortunately, not everyone with significant concerns about ejaculatory control is in a relationship and, in fact, some men might even have avoided becoming involved because of their embarrassment with rapid ejaculation. So, what about the fellow who is currently without a sexual partner. As mentioned above, there is a step-by-step process he can do by himself as he practices solo in anticipation of his next new sexual encounter.

New relationships should not be avoided, as a man will never learn ejaculatory control with a woman if women are shunned. Remember that you will never learn to play golf if you avoid going to the golf course. If a man is looking for an emotional and sexual companion, he will at some point be put to the test. With no first time strategy for coping with these new encounters, he is most likely to be quite apprehensive about those exciting/frightening first times. When the passions mount and the clothes start coming off, both excitement and anxiety skyrocket.

As we have seen, excitement and anxiety will actually contribute to the feared outcome – the uncontrolled rapid ejaculation. If the man is afraid he'll lose control, worries about his partner's disappointment and figures he's going to have to do some serious apologizing, it's obvious the man already knows he'll ejaculate quickly. He probably will.

However, if he has decided he is not going to tell his partner of his prediction, he is allowing her to formulate her own expectations and to build her own hopes of how the encounter will go. She might be looking forward to a prolonged session involving all of her favorite positions, but suddenly and unexpectedly, the man who has aroused her now moans "Oh Shit!" and ejaculates! He knew it would happen, but she didn't and he must now try to explain, apologize or beat himself up to prove to her that he really had intended to be spectacular!

Many men wrap much of their male ego around their image as a competent sexual performer and the thought of admitting to a woman any lack of knowledge or any apprehension about performance is unthinkable. However, I strongly believe that the best strategy for a new experience is to <u>forewarn the unsuspecting woman</u>! It is amazing to me that so many man recoil in shock when I suggest this, and ask me in wide-eyed disbelief, "You mean I've got to admit I have a problem?" . . . as if she's not going to discover it on her own!

I will once more suggest that thinking of rapid ejaculation as a "problem" only contributes to discomfort and loss of sexual self-esteem. I suggest a strategy such as the following. As the excitement mounts and the touching progresses, the man begins to talk. Remember that women usually love *pillow talk*. "I love how you feel . . . you excite me so! I want to make you feel good and to learn everything I can about your fantastic body. I want to know what feels best to you and what works best for you." With this reassurance he has told her of his desire to give her pleasure, and now he will do everything possible to give her all the non-coital pleasure she desires.

"You excite me so much!" he repeats. "I think I am so excited that I probably will not last very long. Let's not worry about me this time, but now just let me give to you. This will be for you, so help me learn how to give you pleasure. I'll get my turn later." When it is time for vaginal penetration, it should not be rushed into and might be best if it follows the woman's orgasm if he has learned she is not orgasmic during intercourse. He should invite her to mount him, starting and stopping as best he can during these early encounters. "Wow, don't move! You are driving me wild! Stay still for a moment. You feel so very very good."

After his orgasm the man offers <u>no apologies</u>. Rather, he should congratulate her. "Wow, that was fantastic for me . . . didn't last long, but you really felt great to me. I just couldn't hold back, but it was wonderful. Next time we'll work on my lasting a bit longer, but right now, I just want to hold you." No Trauma! No Drama!

This is so much more positive than what typically happens when a man has to apologize after the fact! It reassures the woman that his rapid ejaculation was not a selfish act. Remember, many women misinterpret the motives of a man who ejaculates quickly, thinking that was all he had wanted. Talking about it in a positive and playful way opens up the communication about what feels good to this particular woman. Remember, <u>each woman is unique</u> and men are not natural born mind readers. This first-time strategy also introduces the idea of a continuing relationship in which, as a couple, they can talk and work on achieving longer sessions of lovemaking.

Most important is that in forewarning the woman, the man decreases the pressure he would feel to impress her with his control, as he has already admitted his vulnerability. If expectations are clear and optimistic, it is likely there will be additional relaxed and playful encounters.

A FINAL WORD

I will repeat again the need to be patient, for there is no quick way to gain better management of the ejaculatory process. In the course of learning, take advantage of the opportunity to learn all about your partner and help her learn all about you. Be creative in pleasuring her, remembering that intercourse is not always the most effective way to satisfy a woman.

If your partner enjoys being on top, allow her to run things until she is satisfied. For many women, this is the best way for them to experience orgasm during intercourse, and for most men, if they remain passive, it is the best position to monitor their progression. When it's your turn, you can then choose whatever position you prefer.

There is a Chinese proverb that say "Give a man a fish and he'll eat today. Teach a man to fish and he'll eat forever." Learning how to monitor and manage your arousal is like learning how to fish, for once you learn how to manage and delay your ejaculation, the strategy is good forever. As soon as you forget or become too excited, you will quickly find that there has been no real 'cure.' The bad news is that what you learn you must continue to practice, but the good news is that it is a lot of fun!

Remember also that you are the expert at "quickies,"

and there might still be times when your partner offers you an opportunity to have her your way. If she's really not very aroused and is giving you a gift, it is best not to linger too long. In this case, I suspect you will know what to do to just get the job done quickly. Your partner will be appreciative and Mother Nature will be proud.

TENTATIVE SCHEDULE AT A GLANCE

A Recap

At any stage of the homework, it is important not to rush into the next step if you are still feeling anxious, tense, and/or out of control. It is better to take too long than to hurry through the steps and not learn anything about the management of your ejaculatory process!

Schedule your encounters at least twice per week, always planning your session prior to your usual bedtime. Build in showers and perhaps the creation of a romantic and sensual atmosphere.

The following tentative calendar of sessions is meant only as a rough guideline in planning your unique schedule. If you have a partner, always plan with her and in a way that neither of you feel pressured.

Remember that your schedule need not be carved in stone, and can be adjusted as other things come up or as energy levels go down. Also remember that you can treat yourself to an occasional "quickie" with your partner's consent and, if she desires, before or after satisfying her.

❏ **1ˢᵗ & 2ⁿᵈ Week for both**
Nonsexual sensate focus for both, with music, candles and massage oil.

❏ **1ˢᵗ & 2ⁿᵈ Week for him alone**
Between sensate focus sessions with your partner, use start/stop masturbation if necessary.

❏ **3ʳᵈ & 4ᵗʰ Week for her**
Sexual sensate focus with an emphasis on your verbal communication. She receives oral stimulation if both agree. Time to learn what works best for her orgasms.

❏ **3ʳᵈ & 4ᵗʰ Week for him**
After some nonsexual touch, begin slow stimulation of his penis with a dry hand. He remains passive on his back as he focuses on arousal level and starts and stops five or six times.

❏ **4ᵗʰ & 5ᵗʰ Week for her**
More sexual sensate focus, learning what feels best to her. Orgasms as needed. Oral stimulation for her if she likes.

❏ **4ᵗʰ & 5ᵗʰ Week for him**
After starting & stopping two times with dry manual stimulation, stimulation of penis with a lubricated hand and, if OK for both, oral stimulation on him. He focuses on arousal level and starts and stops five or six times.

❏ **5ᵗʰ - 7ᵗʰ Week for her:**
Lots of foreplay for her. Become an expert on what pleases her. Orgasms with manual or oral stimulation if she desires prior to "outercourse."

❏ **5ᵗʰ Week for him**
After relaxing and a couple starts/stops with a lubricated hand, she straddles him with his penis between the lips of her genitals ("outercourse"). She

slides as he keeps track, starting and stopping a total of five or six times. He remains passive, with eyes closed and focusing on his arousal level.

❏ 6th Week for <u>both</u>

She mounts and slides from front to back with more "outercourse." Start and stop five or six times with him passive on his back, but with his eyes open and hand on her hips as he keeps track of arousal level.

❏ 7th Week for <u>both</u>

Mounts as before, but during "outercourse" he allows visual stimulation and rich erotic fantasy, but still keeping track and starting and stopping a total of five or six times

❏ 7th & 8th Week for <u>both</u>

Once he is relaxed and in good control during outercourse, she mounts and inserts his penis, sliding down and sitting quietly until he signals he is back under control. She then moves front to back and he remains passive, relaxed and with eyes closed as he focuses on his level of arousal. Start and stop at least six times.

❏ 9th Week and beyond

Lots of communication and foreplay. Experiment with some new positions and rates of thrusting. He keeps careful track and slows or stops as needed, something he will now do for the rest of his sexual life.

YOUR NOTES:

Do an honest assessment of your thoughts and feelings. Share with a partner or keep private. You might even decide to make a copy and have your partner make her own notes without seeing your responses, and then share. Talking about what you each recorded.

My sexual worries and anxieties:

Things to watch out for:

Things I know or have learned that my partner likes:

Things I am good at in bed:

RAPID EJACULATION SELF ASSESSMENT

Your responses to the following questions might assist you to clarify or to better understand your concerns about premature or rapid ejaculation. Respond to each question as truthfully and completely as you can, answering as you really feel or think, not as you think you should.

1. Is your problem with rapid ejaculation a new one? **(YES) (NO)** If **YES**, when did it seem to start?

_____

_____

2. Is your problem a chronic one [life long] **(YES) (NO)** If **YES**, what have you tried in the past to gain better control?

_____

_____

3. How often are you attempting to have intercourse? _____ Who typically initiates? _____

4. How long does the foreplay typically last before any penetration is made?_____ Is there anything about the type or duration of foreplay that seems to influence your control? **(YES) (NO)** If **YES**, what?_____

_____

5. Do you ever ejaculate just **prior** to penetration? (YES) (NO) If **YES,** what percent of the time?_____%

6. Do you ever ejaculate **immediately** upon penetrating? (YES) (NO) If **YES,** what percent of the time?_____%

7. If you can accomplish penetration, how quickly are you ejaculating once you begin intercourse? _____(minutes) (seconds)

8. What percent of the time do **you** feel you have ejaculated too quickly?_____% What percent of the time does your **partner** think you were too quick?_____%

9. Do you ever get a second erection and ejaculate a second time? (YES) (NO) If **YES,** how often does this occur?_____ If you are able to experience a second ejaculation, how long can you last once intercourse begins this second time?_____ (seconds) (minutes)

10. Do you masturbate? (YES) (NO) If **YES,** how often?_____(per week)(month). How long are you lasting with this **self**-stimulation?_____(seconds)(minutes) If you control your ejaculation during masturbation, how are you doing this?_____

_____

_____

11. Is you partner comfortable stimulating you manually during foreplay? (**YES**) (**NO**) If **YES**, how long do you last with your **partner's** manual stimulation?_____ (seconds) (minutes). If you are lasting longer than with intercourse, try to explain why! _____

_____

_____

_____

12. Is your partner comfortable with giving oral stimulation? (**YES**) (**NO**) If **YES**, how long do you last when orally stimulated?_____ (seconds) (minutes). If you are lasting longer with oral stimulation than with intercourse, try to explain why! _____

_____

_____

_____

13. During foreplay, do you worry about ejaculating with this preliminary touching? (**YES**) (**NO**) Do you worry about ejaculating too rapidly before even beginning foreplay? (**YES**) (**NO**) Is there anything about your level of anxiety or stress that seems to influence your control?

_____

_____

_____

_____

14. How often do you desire sex?_____ (per week) (per month)   How often does your partner desire_____ (per week) (per month) Do you ever avoid initiating sex because of a fear of ejaculating too rapidly? (**YES**) (**NO**) If **YES**, how frequent is this?_____ (per week) (per month)

15. Are you experiencing any problems obtaining or maintaining an erection? (**YES**) (**NO**) If **YES**, do you ever ejaculate rapidly even though your penis is not hard? (**YES**) (**NO**)   Do you ever ejaculate even before you feel fully aroused? (**YES**) (**NO**)

16. Does the position of intercourse make a difference in your ability to last? (**YES**) (**NO**) If **YES**, what positions work best?_____
If you last longer in some positions of intercourse, what do you think the difference is? _____

_____

_____

_____

17. Do you have more than one partner? (**YES**) (**NO**) If **YES**, can you last longer with one than with another? (**YES**) (**NO**)   If **YES**, what do you think the difference is?

_____

_____

_____

_____

18. What is your reaction when you ejaculate rapidly?

_____

_____

_____

_____

19. What is your partner(s) reaction when it happens?

_____

_____

_____

_____

20. Are you bringing your partner to orgasm before you ejaculate, or after?_____ If neither, why not?

_____

_____

_____

Does everything stop once you have ejaculated? (**YES**) (**NO**) If **YES**, who wants to stop? (You) (Your partner) (Both)

21. What have you attempted in the past to gain better control or to last longer?_____

_____

_____

_____

Has anything seemed to help? (**YES**) (**NO**) If **YES**, what?

_____

_____

_____

22. Has any partner compared you with another lover, e.g., "He could last an hour, why can't you?" **(YES) (NO)** Has any partner questioned your love, e.g., "If you loved me you would last longer to satisfy me." **(YES) (NO)** If **YES**, how have you reacted? _____

_____

_____

_____

23. Has any partner attempted to reassure you, e.g., "It doesn't matter," or "I loved all the rest of it." **(YES) (NO)** If **YES**, how have you reacted? _____

_____

_____

_____

24. Do you believe that your rapid ejaculation is a physical problem, a psychological problem, or a combination of both? _____
Thoughts? _____

25. Have you sought help for this concern in the past? **(YES)(NO)** If **YES**, what was recommended and what did you try? _____

_____

_____

_____

26. Have you read another self-help book by another author? **(YES) (NO)** If **YES**, what similarities did you find?

_____

_____

_____

_____

_____

What differences? _____

_____

_____

_____

_____

Add any thoughts or insights:

_____

_____

_____

_____

_____

_____

_____

_____

_____

_____

_____

_____

_____

If you are seeing a counselor or therapist about your ejaculatory concern, after completing this questionnaire, take it to your next appointment.

PROFESSIONAL RESOURCES

If you find that you are unable to gain satisfactory control on your own or if your relationship is in serious trouble because of your rapid ejaculation or other sexual concerns, do not hesitate to consult a **qualified** sexuality therapist or counselor. If there are no other relationship issues, a well trained and experienced sex therapist can assist you in a relatively brief period of time. To locate a qualified professional in your geographic area, write to one or both of the following national certificating associations:

American Academy of Clinical Sexologists
3203 Lawton Road, Suite 170
Orlando, FL 32803
(407) 645-1641   http://www.esextherapy.com

American Association of Sex Educators, Counselors and Therapists
P.O. Box 1960
Ashland, VA 23005-1960
(804) 644-3288   http://www.aasect.org

BOOK AND MEDIA RESOURCES

Birch, R. W. (1997) *MALE SEXUAL ENDURANCE: A Man's Book About Ejaculatory Control*, 8" X 10" with photo illustrations.

YOU CAN LAST LONGER DVD, hosted by Dr. Derek C. Polonsky of the Harvard Medical School and Dr. Marian E. Dunn, certified sex therapist. Volume 8 of The Better Sex Video Series.

The above books and DVD are available from the website at http://www.oralcaress.com or by writing to PEC Publishing, 429 Grand Ridge Drive, Howard, OH 43028

Helen Singer Kaplan (1987) *PE: HOW TO OVERCOME PREMATURE EJACULATION* (Available through http://www.amazon.com)

Michael E. Metz and Barry W. McCarthy (2003) *COPING WITH PREMATURE EJACULATION* (Available through http://www.amazon.com)

ABOUT THE AUTHOR

Robert Birch, Ph.D. had specialized in marital, family and sex therapy for over 30 years. Dr. Birch received his Bachelor's Degree in psychology in 1960 from Muskingum College, his Master's Degree in psychology in 1962 from The University of Ohio, and his Ph.D. in Psychology from The University of Wisconsin in 1967. He had been a sex therapy consultant to the Medical Center at Wright-Patterson Air Force Base, had been an adjunct faculty member in The Ohio State University Family Therapy program, and had served on the national board of directors of the American Association for Marriage and Family Therapy (AAMFT), the American Association of Sex Educators, Counselors and Therapists (AASECT), and the Board of Examiners of the American Board of Family Psychology.

Dr. Birch had been certified by AASECT as a Sex Therapist, as a Sex Educator and as a Supervisor and was a Clinical Member, a Fellow and an Approved Supervisor of AAFMT. He was certified as a Family Therapist by the National Alliance of Certified Family Therapists, and was certified as a Sex Therapist and a Supervisor by the American Board of Sexology. During his years of practice, Dr. Birch had been named a Founding Fellow of the American Academy of Clinical Sexologists, a Fellow of the American Academy of Family Psychology, and a Diplomate of the American Board of Family Psychology.

Dr. Birch has presented over 350 guest lectures and led over 100 professional workshops and seminars. During his professional career he had served as the Audio-Visual Review Editor of the *Journal of Sex Education and Therapy,* as well as having been on the Editorial Board of that journal and of the *Journal of Family Therapy.* He has written eight books, co-authored one book, and co-authored a chapter on female sexuality for a book on women's health issues.

Dr. Birch retired from practice in 1998 after 35 years as a psychologist. In his retirement, Dr. Birch has moved to rural Ohio where he continues to write in the company of his wife and four dogs.

OTHER SELF-HELP BOOKS BY THE AUTHOR

ORAL CARESS: The Loving Guide to Exciting a Woman
1-57074-307-X, 1996

CUNNILINGUS: Warm Her Heart and Tickle Her Pink
1-57074-500-5, 2006

A SEX THERAPIST'S MANUAL: Resources for Clinical or Educational Use 1-57074-320-7, 1996

MALE SEXUAL ENDURANCE: A Man's Book about Ejaculatory Control 1-57074-349-5, 1997

SENSUAL PATHWAYS TO PLEASURE: A Woman's Journey to Orgasm, Coauthored by Cynthia Lief Ruberg, 2006

SEX AND THE AGING MALE: Understanding and Coping with Change 1-57074-482-3, 2000

TOO BIG: A Guide for When Pain Replaces Pleasure,
1-44951-979-2, 2009

These books are available from the author's website at www.oralcaress.com.

www.ingramcontent.com/pod-product-compliance
Lightning Source LLC
Chambersburg PA
CBHW062111280526
45788CB00003B/1440